THE BASIC NEW YEAR LIFE GOALS

Guides to Setting your Health & Wellness Fitness Goals (2023)

NORA U.I

Contents

INTRODUCTION

Unbelievably, the term "wellness" used to be more commonly associated with natural food markets and vitamin advertisements. In reality, for a very long time, exercise was prioritized over wellness simply because it was more hip and exciting, especially from a marketing standpoint. That is obviously no longer the case. Consumers are looking for ways to create balance in a time when life seems to be moving at an exponential rate and schedules are jam-packed to the brim, and the wellness sector is booming as a result. Let's examine why wellness merits special attention from both consumers and professionals, even though physical fitness will always be at the core of the work of health and exercise specialists.

Fitness is the ability to perform physical tasks or the absence of physical ailments. It specifically refers to physical health. Contrarily, wellness is the state of having a variety of aspects of one's life that are in harmony with regard to one's health. The majority of wellness wheels include the intellectual, emotional, physical, occupational, environmental, spiritual, social, and financial elements of wellness as well as six to seven more components. All of the aforementioned aspects of life are taken into account and given priority in everyday lifestyle habits when a person is balanced and healthy.

The idea of personal balance and whole-person wellbeing has gained popularity. Clients seek a more holistic and wellness-based service when they consult with health and fitness professionals. This is not meant to minimize the value of physical activity and general fitness. Getting into a workout routine is frequently the first step in improving one's health. Once customers develop wholesome exercise routines, they frequently feel confident and motivated to investigate other aspects of fitness.

CHAPTER ONE

Goals are what for?

Why Are Goals Set?

Even the most diligent labor is eventually reduced to little more than a necessary interruption between weekends in the absence of clear, explicit goals.

Goals help focus energy. By outlining what must be done and establishing reasonable time constraints for it, goals can help you perform at your best. Obstacles are essentially the basis of our successes when it comes to bringing out true triumphs.

Goals provide guidance One might use the cliché of traveling without a destination to grasp the significance of goals. Depending on where you are on your trip, it can even make you happy. Does it still make sense if you aren't on vacation, though? Definitely not! The same is true for objectives. You choose the destination and the time frame, and the route is automatically decided for you. Once the route is chosen, you may confirm that you are on course and within the allotted time.

An Approach to Goal Setting in Steps:

The following are the key considerations while setting a goal.

Setting goals is a continuous process of self-discovery.

No matter what anyone has said about you or your abilities, you can use your inner vision to see things that others might not have been able to. In every area of your life, the chipping away can be a continuous process of self-discovery and success. You have numerous opportunities to design a life that is consistent with the objectives you have established for yourself, as opposed to Michelangelo, who only had one chance to carve that enormous block of marble.

Understanding Your Passion

Four fundamental questions should be addressed.

What would I really love to do with my life if time, money, and personal responsibilities weren't constraints? In other words, what would you start doing the next day if you could start doing whatever you wanted? You can better define your response by answering the other three questions.

What activities did you like as a child? Or what possessed you as a true expert? What caused you to feel admired?

Why do you feel that way right now?

Are you making an effort to help others? Does that make you feel proud of yourself and successful?

Norms for Goals-Setting

Dream big and never give up.

Positive and negative beliefs are two distinct categories. The key to unlocking the door to success for every person is a positive belief expressed as a goal. Negative beliefs, on the other hand, are the mental barriers that may keep us from success for good.

Clearly state your objective:

Be clear about your goals for both your personal and professional life. You ought to be able to elaborate on your plan. Set your own target date in order to attain the goal. Make a strategy for achieving your goal step by step.

Try your hardest to win:

Most individuals frame their thinking around an eight-hour day. You must be doing something no one else is doing to succeed.

Continue to be flexible:

Change is ongoing and continuous. Individuals and organizations with stiff structures are prone to being carried away easily.

However, those people and corporate cultures that shift quickly survive and prosper. As you go forward along your chosen course, it is crucial to remain on the lookout for fresh chances.

SUCCESSFUL FITNESS RESOLUTIONS FOR THE NEW YEAR

LEARN SMART

Implementing the (SMART) system, a five-step process that can keep you focused and on track, can help you avoid feeling overwhelmed when setting goals. The letters in the acronym stand for time-based, relevant, particular, measurable, and achievable outcome. You may need to reconsider how achievable your goals are and think about changing them if they don't fall into those categories.

By the end of the year, you can attain even the most ambitious goals, such as the nine we've outlined, if you're able to lock and load your goals into the (SMART). Formula

The majority of people make exercise and health goals as part of their New Year's resolutions every year, but many of them are not kept.

A person may not succeed in achieving a goal for a number of reasons, such as a lack of long-term persistence, a lack of conscious action, or outright forgetfulness.

1. Think about your Why.

Consider the reasons you chose your goal and why they are significant to you. When motivation wanes, remembering why you established the goal will inspire you to complete it.

2. Make sure your objectives are quantifiable.

Once a goal has been established, be sure it can also be measured so you can carefully and consistently track your progress. Make sure your effort is in accordance with the results you are aiming to attain. Sometimes, a re-calibration, a plan modification, or an adjustment may be required.

3. Be Specific and Narrow Down.

Setting too many fitness goals is the biggest error athletes make. Focus on the one or two objectives that are most essential to you at this time, and work toward achieving them until you are ready to move on to something else.

4. Develop Self-Control.

Every time we establish a goal, we must make an effort that is different from what we usually do, which calls for self-control. Use the neuron training activities on Rewire to start practicing self-control and developing mental resilience.

5. Establish reasonable but challenging goals.

Make sure the objectives you set are challenging but doable. They shouldn't be impossible for you to complete, but they also shouldn't be impossible for you. You'll feel great once you've completed them, and you'll be ready to set new ones.

6. Increase your sense of self-worth.

In Bandura's (1997) Social-Cognitive Theory, self-efficacy is your confidence in your capacity to carry out specific tasks. Psychological research has demonstrated that increasing one's self-efficacy improves performance, attention, concentration, effort, and optimism in the face of obstacles.

You can use visualization as a powerful technique to get ready and succeed in reaching your fitness goals.

CHAPTER TWO

Just keep it basic

Healthy nutrition to obtain fitness

1. Avoid sugary beverages.

The main source of added sugar in the American diet is sweetened beverages like soda, fruit juice, and tea.

Sadly, research from multiple studies indicates that even in people who do not have extra body fat, drinking sugar-sweetened beverages increases the risk of type 2 diabetes and heart disease.

Sugar-sweetened beverages are particularly detrimental for kids since they can cause illnesses including type 2 diabetes, high blood pressure, and non-alcoholic fatty liver disease, which typically do not manifest in children until maturity, in addition to obesity in kids.

Alternatives that are healthier include:

1. Water
2. Teas without sugar
3. Frothy water
4. Coffee

2. Consume seeds and nuts.

The high fat content of nuts causes some people to shun them. However, nuts and seeds are highly healthy. They include a wealth of vitamins, minerals, fiber, and protein.

Nuts may aid in weight loss and lower your risk of heart disease and type 2 diabetes.

A significant observational study also found a possible connection between a low diet of nuts and seeds and a higher risk of dying from heart disease, stroke, or type 2 diabetes.

3. Steer clear of highly processed meals.

Foods with ingredients that have undergone extensive modification from their original state are considered ultra-processed. Added sugar, highly refined oil, salt, preservatives, artificial sweeteners, colors, and flavors are among the additives that are frequently included in them.

Examples comprise:

1. Snack cakes

2. Quick meals

3. Freeze-dried foodstuffs

4. Foods in cans
5. Chips

Ultra-processed foods are highly delicious, which makes them easy to overeat, and they activate reward-related brain regions, which might result in an excessive intake of calories and weight gain. According to studies, eating a lot of ultra-processed foods can increase your risk of developing chronic diseases like type 2 diabetes, heart disease, and obesity.

4. Consume oily fish.

A fantastic source of high-quality protein and good fat is fish. The anti-inflammatory omega-3 fatty acids and other nutrients found in fatty fish like salmon make this especially true.

According to studies, people who regularly consume fish have a lower risk of developing a number of diseases, such as heart disease, dementia, and inflammatory bowel disease.

5. Get adequate rest.

It is impossible to stress the significance of obtaining adequate quality sleep.

Poor sleep can drive insulin resistance, upset your appetite hormones, and diminish your physical and mental function.

Additionally, getting too little sleep is a weak individual risk factor for weight gain and obesity. People who get enough sleep don't prefer to choose foods that are higher in calories, fat, and sugar, which could result in unintended weight gain.

6. Keep hydrated.

Hydration is a crucial yet frequently disregarded indicator of health. Maintaining enough blood volume and good physiological function are both made possible by being hydrated.

The best approach to staying hydrated is to drink water, which has no calories, sugar, or chemicals.

Although there isn't a fixed amount that everyone requires each day, try to drink enough to adequately quench your thirst.

7. Consume a lot of fruits and vegetables.

Prebiotic fiber, vitamins, minerals, and antioxidants, many of which have powerful health benefits, are abundant in fruits and vegetables.

According to studies, those who consume more fruits and vegetables generally live longer and are at a decreased risk of developing heart disease, obesity, and other diseases.

8. Consume enough protein.

Consuming adequate protein will help you stay healthy since it gives your body the building blocks it needs to make new cells and tissues.

Additionally, this substance is crucial for maintaining a healthy body weight. While making you feel full, a high-protein diet may increase your metabolic rate, or the rate at which calories are burned. Additionally, it might lessen your need to nibble late at night and curb cravings.

9. Move forward

One of the best things you can do for your mental and physical health is to engage in aerobic exercise, or cardio.

It works especially well at shedding belly fat, the unhealthy kind of fat that collects around your organs.

Do exercises that help you become in shape.

Most people have a tendency to concentrate on one sort of exercise or activity and believe that this is sufficient. According to research, exercise should include all four types: endurance, strength, balance, and flexibility. Each one offers various advantages. The ability to perform one sort can also help you perform the others better, and variation lowers boredom and injury risk. Whatever your age, you can find activities to suit your needs and physical level.

Exercises for young and older people's endurance

Your breathing and heart rate rise when you engage in endurance exercises, also known as aerobic exercises. With the help of these exercises, you can maintain your health, improve your fitness, and carry out your daily responsibilities. The health of your heart, lungs, and circulatory system are all improved by endurance training. They also have the power to postpone or even reverse several illnesses that are common in older people, including diabetes, breast and colon cancer, heart disease, and others. Exercises that increase endurance include:

Dancing, swimming, biking, climbing stairs or hills, playing tennis or basketball, brisk walking or jogging, yard work (mowing, raking), and other activities are examples of physical activities.

In order to keep up with your grandchildren on a park stroll, dance to your favorite tunes at a family wedding, and rake and bag leaves, you should increase your endurance, or "staying power." Build up to performing vigorous exercise for at least 150 minutes per week. To achieve this goal, make an effort to stay active during the day and avoid spending too much time sitting down.

Safety advice

Warm up and cool down by performing a brief, easy exercise, like brisk walking, before and after your endurance exercises.

Pay attention to your body; endurance exercises shouldn't make you feel lightheaded, anxious, or as though you have heartburn.

When engaging in any activity that causes you to perspire, remember to hydrate. Before increasing the amount of fluid you consume while exercising, make sure to check with your doctor if they have advised you to limit your fluid intake.

Be mindful of your surroundings if you plan to exercise outside.

Wear layers so you can add or take away clothing as the temperature changes.

Use safety gear, such as a helmet when biking, to prevent accidents.

Age-appropriate strength training

Your muscular power can significantly impact the situation. Strong muscles help you maintain your independence and make simple tasks like getting out of a chair, climbing stairs, and carrying groceries feel simpler. Keeping your muscles healthy can improve your balance and help you avoid falls and injuries associated with falls. When your hip and leg muscles are strong, you are less prone to tripping and falling. Strength training or "resistance training" are two terms used to describe the process of utilizing weights to increase muscle strength.

Some people decide to use weights to increase their strength. If so, begin with small weights and progressively increase them. Others employ resistance bands, which are supple elastic bands with different strengths. If you're just starting out, work out without the band at first or only use a little band until you feel comfortable. When you can complete two sets of 10 to 15 repetitions without difficulty, you can add a band or upgrade to a stronger band (or more weight). Try to perform strength training for each of your major muscle groups at least twice a week. Avoid working out the same muscle twice in a row, however. Here are a few illustrations of strength training:

Lifting weights, carrying groceries, gripping a tennis ball, overhead arm curls, arm curls, and wall push-ups are some examples of exercises.

Lifting your own body weight and applying a resistance band

Safety advice

While doing strength training, breathe normally and avoid holding your breath.

As you raise or push, exhale, and as you relax, inhale.

If you have any questions regarding a particular workout, consult your doctor.

When you can complete two sets of 10 to 15 repetitions without difficulty, you can add a band or upgrade to a stronger band (or more weight). Try to perform strength training for each of your major muscle groups at least twice a week; however, avoid working out the same muscle twice in a row. Here are a few illustrations of strength training:

Lifting weights, carrying groceries, gripping a tennis ball, overhead arm curls, arm curls, and wall push-ups are some examples of exercises.

Lifting your own body weight and applying a resistance band

Safety advice

While doing strength training, breathe normally and avoid holding your breath.

As you raise or push, exhale, and as you relax, inhale.

If you have any questions regarding a particular workout, consult your doctor.

CHAPTER THREE

Physical health and wellbeing

An individual's level of physical fitness reflects their overall health, particularly their social, mental, emotional, and spiritual wellbeing. The physical aspect of wellness promotes regular physical activity as well as cardiovascular flexibility and strength. The promotion of physical development discourages the use of tobacco, narcotics, and excessive alcohol use while encouraging understanding of nutrition and diet.

Physical wellness promotes behaviors and consumption that support high levels of wellness, such as medical self-care and sensible use of the healthcare system. You'll aim to spend more time each week developing your physical strength, flexibility, and endurance as you move along the path to physical wellness. The path may occasionally grow narrow and dangerous; as a result, you'll become more conscious of the dangers in your immediate environment and start to take preventative measures to ensure your safe passage. In order to be physically healthy, one must be able to take care of minor illnesses on one's own and recognize when seeking professional medical help is necessary.

You will be able to monitor your own vital signs and recognize your body's warning signs by physically following the path of wellness. You'll comprehend and value the link between healthy eating and how your body functions. The physical aspect of wellbeing yields both physical and psychological benefits almost immediately. The psychological advantages of improved self-esteem, self-control, determination, and a sense of direction are frequently a result of the physical advantages of looking great and feeling fantastic.

Physical wellness includes activities that you must engage in to maintain your health. The combination of beneficial physical activity/exercise and healthy eating habits leads to the development of optimal physical wellness. Building muscular strength and endurance, cardiovascular strength and endurance, and flexibility are essential elements of physical wellness.

The development of personal responsibility for your own health care, including the ability to treat minor ailments on your own and recognize when you require expert medical assistance, is another aspect of physical wellbeing. By improving your physical wellness, you have the ability to keep track of your own vital signs and recognize your body's warning indications. You'll comprehend and value the link between healthy eating and how your body functions.

The psychological advantages of higher self-esteem and self-control are frequently a result of the physical advantages of looking great and feeling great.

ESSENTIAL ELEMENTS OF FITNESS:

The following are the four main factors (also known as the health-related fitness factors) that are crucial for bettering physical health:

• Cardio respiratory capacity is the body's capability to breathe in air, transport it to cells, and utilize it to produce energy in cells (bioenergetics) for physical activity (activity). Cardio-respiratory capacity is also referred to as aerobic capacity in the fitness industry. This ability encompasses aerobic strength, aerobic power, and aerobic endurance (how long it lasts) (how fast) Cardiopulmonary exercise can reduce resting heart rate, lower risk of cardiovascular disease, enhance endurance, raise stroke volume, and boost cardiac output, to name a few long-term adaptations.

The range of muscular capability is referred to as muscular capacity. This includes muscular strength, which is the capacity to generate force or the maximum amount of force that a muscle can exert in a single contraction; muscular endurance, which is the capacity to apply force over a prolonged period of time or to complete repeated muscle contractions; and muscular power (i.e. the ability to generate strength in an explosive way). The enhanced strength, greater muscular endurance, increased basal metabolic rate, improved joint strength, and overall posture are some of the long-term adaptations of increased muscular capacity.

The amount of motion or range of motion that a joint is capable of performing is known as flexibility. Different joints have varying degrees of flexibility. A few long-term adaptations of increased flexibility include a lower chance of injury, an expanded range of motion, and better posture.

• The ratio of fat-free mass (muscle, bone, blood, organs, and fluids) to total body mass is known as body composition (adipose tissue deposited under the skin and around organs). Decreased risk of cardiovascular disease, increased basal metabolic rate, enhanced physiological function, and improved BMI are a few long-term adaptations of altering body composition.

SECONDARY FITNESS COMPONENTS

All physical activity involves the secondary components of fitness, which are often referred to as the performance-based fitness components. These components are essential for daily functioning. Depending on how well these ancillary fitness components are developed, athletes achieve varying degrees of success. We shouldn't overlook the secondary components of fitness because they are crucial to completing daily chores, even though the basic components are regarded to be the most crucial. The following are the secondary components.

• The ability to maintain a particular body position in either a static or dynamic (moving) situation is known as balance.

• The capacity to use all of the body's elements in unison to create fluid, smooth movements is known as coordination.

Ability is the capacity to quickly shift course.

The amount of time needed to react to a certain stimuli is known as reaction time.

• The capacity to move quickly is known as speed. Another name for speed is velocity (rate of motion)

• Strength and speed combine to create power. Another name for power is explosive strength.

• Mental capability includes the capacity to relax and take pleasure in the psychological advantages of activity, as well as the capacity to focus while exercise to enhance training results (endorphins).

HAPPINESS AND HEALTH

Due to its constant change, health is a dynamic process. Everyone has periods of excellent health, sickness, and sometimes even major illness. Our level of health changes along with our way of life.

Those of us who engage in regular physical activity do so in part to raise our level of health both now and in the future. We work to achieve the highest possible level of wellbeing. As our way of life improves, so does our health, and we suffer from illness and disease less frequently? When asked what it means to be healthy, the majority of people often list the previously listed four elements of fitness (cardio respiratory ability, muscular ability, flexibility, and body composition). Despite the fact that these elements are essential to good health, they are not the only ones.

Our total health includes more than just our physical wellness.

• Social health - The capacity to successfully interact with others, the environment, and to form fulfilling personal connections.

Ability to study and advance intellectually is a sign of good mental health. Both real-world experiences and more formal institutions (like schools) improve mental health.

• Emotional wellness - The capacity to regulate emotions so that you feel at ease expressing them and can do so in the right circumstances.

A belief in a unifying power is a sign of spiritual wellness. Although it differs from person to person, at its core is the idea of faith.

The pursuit of improved quality of life, personal development, and potential through healthy lifestyle practices and attitudes is known as wellness. Daily health improvements are possible if we accept responsibility for our own health and wellbeing. Our level of wellness is influenced by specific elements. Including excellent nutrition, exercise, stress management techniques, fulfilling relationships, and professional achievement.

To live long, fulfilling lives that are healthy, we strive every day to achieve our highest level of health and wellness. Living a balanced life is essential for the pursuit of health, personal development, and increased quality of life. We must take good care of our mind, body, and soul in order to achieve equilibrium.

We won't be at our healthiest if any of these three areas are neglected or persistently neglected. All through life, finding a balance in each of these three areas is an ongoing challenge.

As fitness experts, it is our duty to mentor and inspire others to increase their level of wellness and health. We may encourage not just physical activity but a comprehensive approach to wellness (mind, body, and spirit). We should set a good example by adopting healthy habits that contribute to both our own and others' wellbeing. If all of our attention is devoted to the physical advantages of exercise, we are failing our clients and failing to uphold our professional duty.

PERKS OF MODERATE ACTIVITY:

As fitness experts, we devote a lot of time to encouraging and aiding others in their quest for better health. Education is a crucial component of this. We must educate individuals about the advantages of regular exercise and the need of staying active.

ACTIVITY RECOMMENDS:

To assist Canadians in making informed decisions about physical exercise as a means of enhancing their health, Health Canada developed the Canada's Physical Activity Guide to Healthy Active Living. According to science, you should engage in 60 minutes of physical activity each day to maintain or enhance your health. The Physical Activity Guide makes the following recommendations:

• Endurance: Engage in continuous action for your heart, lungs, and circulatory system four to seven days a week. Improvements take time, depending on your efforts.

• Flexibility: To maintain muscles relaxed and joints mobile, gently bend, reach, and stretch four to seven days a week.

Strengthen your muscles, bones, and posture by engaging in resistance training two to four days a week.

Additionally, the American College of Sports Medicine (ACSM) has created activity recommendations for enhancing health:

• For cardiovascular health, engage in moderate-intensity exercise for at least 30 minutes each day. The 30-minute period doesn't have to be continuous.

• To maintain and improve muscle strength and endurance, resistance training for 1 set of 8–12 repetitions for the complete body is required.

• In order to preserve mobility, flexibility exercise should be done every day, including stretches for tall major muscle groups.

CHAPTER FOUR

CONCULUSION

How to start and reach your fitness objectives

You could believe that beginning a fitness and health journey is overwhelming. Your mind immediately conjures up a picture of a piece of workout equipment or of someone staring at you. Although it might seem scary, remember that everyone was once a novice.

Making the choice to give up bad behaviors and adopt healthier ones can change your life. Not only will this significantly enhance your general well-being, but it can also enhance your mood, boost your self-confidence, and keep you motivated to stay on course.

We've laid out some tactics to get you started since coming prepared with the appropriate game plan can help you succeed!

1. Choose your cause and make the commitment.

When beginning something, it's important to think about why you're doing it in the first place. Doing it for others or for yourself what do you anticipate gaining from it?

Instead of something you believe you need, it should be something you want. The motivation could be as straightforward as boosting your mental health or not wanting to be out of breath when climbing stairs.

It is ineffective to try to establish a regular exercise schedule, look into the most efficient techniques, or perform other time-consuming duties. Whether or not you're prepared to change is entirely up to you, but if you're not fully dedicated to the procedure, you won't be able to accomplish your goals.

No matter how difficult or challenging it will be, reassure yourself that you are capable of handling anything and everything that may happen.

2. Create a strategy and organize a vision board.

Any goal requires a plan because, while creating a strategy, you need to know what objectives you want to attain and when you want to break them. Establishing your ideal schedule, whether for meditation, meals, or exercise, is crucial.

A vision board often consists of a list with both written and visual elements. It enables you to see your objective, your path, and the strategies you'll need to get there.

Make a vision board so you can begin strategizing and working toward your fitness goals. You can use a shadow box, poster board, bulletin board, or even just a notebook. It shouldn't resemble anyone else's; it should be what motivates you. You could use the following examples to create your fitness vision board:

- Old photographs of you

- Images of wholesome foods

- Short tales of inspiration

- Journal excerpts

- Anything that demonstrates your drive

Put your vision board in a location that you will view it frequently. You may even create a new vision board to reflect your accomplishments.

3. Creating Optimistic and Realistic Goals

Some people desire to increase their stamina, health, and self-assurance. But how do you proceed to get there?

Fitness objectives are crucial for a number of reasons. They hold us responsible, broaden our perspective of the possibilities, and inspire us to push past momentary difficulties in order to make enduring improvements.

While having a huge, overarching objective is important, you should also set more realistic, smaller fitness goals to help you get there.

We all seek instant gratification, but it's critical to set a realistic timetable and keep in mind that everything takes time. Major renovations never get finished in a week.

Choose a goal that you can complete over the course of months as opposed to a year, such as increasing your exercise or watching what you eat. In this sense, if you approach it with a long-term mindset rather than a fast cure mentality, you are more likely to remain with it.

4. Begin with little steps

It is best to gradually increase your level of fitness. You don't need to run a marathon or lift weights on Day 1; otherwise, you risk getting hurt and losing motivation.

Establish a daily cardio routine with your AI Smart Bike for 15 to 30 minutes to develop a regular fitness habit. You can gradually increase the difficulty of your workout programs.

5. Investigate a variety of options to see what suits you best.

To be enthusiastic about your exercise regimen, you must be aware of your preferences. New fashions, entertaining fitness DVDs, and gear are available every year.

To get the most enjoyment out of your workouts, experiment whenever you can and identify your fitness preferences.

Whatever you decide, make sure to arrange time for strength, cardio, and high-intensity training.

6. Monitor Your Development

To ensure that you remain motivated, it's crucial to keep track of your fitness improvement.

7. Maintain Healthy Routines

Healthy habits must be practiced consistently if you want to reach your goals. These routines can be as simple as using your AI Smart Bike three times a week for a 30-minute workout and treating it like a ritual.

Make sure your daily routine includes healthy practices that will help you get the results you want. Making these habits simple will enable you to incorporate them into your daily routine consistently.

In order to create your perfect daily routine, trying to combine too many things at once can be detrimental and counterproductive. It's critical to keep in mind that maintaining good health is a way of life, not a Band-Aid.

Integration of healthy practices can include things like cutting back on screen time and improving sleep. It will help you recuperate from your workouts and will improve your mood every day.

Start with one to three action plans, and if you can maintain them consistently, add more.

Eat a Balanced Diet.

Fitness goes beyond just physical activities. In order to fuel your workouts, you must also make sure that your body is receiving the right nutrients.

When you quickly incorporate the quantity of calories you expend into your eating habits, it doesn't matter. But as time passes, the caloric quality of the food you're eating will matter more and more.

False fats, sweets, artificial colors, and flavorings, among other things, can impair your immunity, increase your chance of getting sick, and prevent the synthesis of hormones that help you burn fat.

Learning which meals will help you stick to your goals will make it easier for you to develop straightforward healthy eating habits and incorporate them into your daily routine. This is the best way to start eating healthily at home.

There's no need to follow the newest diet craze. Start by eating an assortment of fruits and vegetables, along with protein, complex carbohydrates, and healthy fats.

9. Prefer water to carbonated beverages

When you begin a daily regimen and routine activity, you will typically need to drink more water. It's a signal from your body that you shouldn't disregard!

Drinking enough water before, during, and after any activity is referred to as hydrating. Your body stays cold, and your joints stay lubricated. Water enhances the distribution of nutrients, keeping you healthy and energized.

Lack of appropriate hydration impairs your body's ability to function, which can cause major side effects like muscle cramps, fatigue, and disorientation.

Recharge and hydrate, especially if you frequently engage in strenuous exercise. Water consumption is equally as crucial as healthy food.

10. Avoid letting your cheat days undo your accomplishments.

Cheat days are acceptable as long as you use caution. A tiny piece of cake is acceptable, but don't overindulge or you'll undo all your hard work.

You can love your fitness program even more and keep reaping the benefits for the rest of your life by balancing workouts with healthy nutrition and a life filled with the odd indulgence.

11. Locate a workout partner

It might be intimidating to begin your fitness journey, but having a support system can be helpful. They may support and encourage one another while having fun. In the end, having a reliable workout partner boosts your likelihood of sticking to your routine!

12. Expect Challenges

Life frequently throws you curveballs. You might discover that you are too busy with job, your family, or life in general to put in as much work as you would want.

Everyone has been in the situation when they adhere to their diet for a week before breaking it with a weekend heist. You make a commitment to work out more, work out for three days, but after a long day at work, you struggle to get out of bed.

You develop job aspirations and are mesmerized by the opportunities, only to be bogged down by day-to-day obligations and lack the energy for exercise for several weeks or months.

Try a different training method to see which one you prefer if you're having difficulties keeping motivated to workout. Make a plan in advance to prevent losing motivation at the last minute if you're concerned about it. To stay motivated and remind yourself of why you're doing it, find some inspiring quotes.

The most crucial thing is to persist. Come back as soon as you can. Find little ways to move more throughout the day. Remember that exercise is always preferable to none.

13. Value Recovery Days

The amount of time and effort you put into your workouts and your recovery time are both crucial. The muscles are under a lot of strain with every workout. You need to allow yourself enough time to recuperate after exercise because it puts a lot of strain on your body in order to continue exercising. Try to limit the number of days you work out to three, and then give yourself at least one day to recover between sessions.

14. Put sleep first

Those who wish to reach their objectives must commit to getting enough rest. Taking care of your health is important for reaching goals.

You can be getting less sleep as a result of other commitments like job or business. Create a sleeping routine that will allow you to receive 7 to 9 hours per night of sleep, and plan your activities around it.

For the muscles to recover correctly from workouts and build strength, sleep is particularly crucial.

Your capacity to think clearly will deteriorate if you only get a few hours of sleep each night, making it more difficult for you to accomplish your goals. Take advantage of sleep's profoundly restorative abilities for your body and mind.

The importance of taking breaks and getting enough sleep cannot be overstated. But make sure you're getting enough sleep so you can recharge and continue working toward your objectives.

Remember that just because you start a fitness regimen doesn't mean you have to quit doing everything else. For the majority of people, maintaining a balance is the key to fitness and health. Take occasional breaks for yourself!

When it comes to health, it's important to find a hobby you enjoy while keeping an open mind, so be flexible and modify what you dislike. You need perseverance and tenacity if you want to succeed. You must always keep in mind to be nice and kind to oneself.

Now that you know how to begin your fitness adventure, why not get started right away? You'll accomplish a lot before the year is up.

www.ingramcontent.com/pod-product-compliance
Lightning Source LLC
LaVergne TN
LVHW020531160826
845677LV00015B/3999

* 9 7 9 8 3 5 1 7 4 3 2 4 0 *